MW01264817

MIGRAINE JOURNAL

©2016 Anneline Sophia

www.annelinesophiadesigns.com

DATE: _____

SEVERITY SCALE: 1 2 3 4 5 6 7 8 9 10

SYMPTOMS:
LIGHT SENSITIVITY: _   NAUSEA: _
SICKNESS: _   DIZZINESS: _
OTHER:_____

DURATION: _____

MEDICATION BEFORE MIGRAINE: _____
MEDICATION DURING MIGRAINE: _____
TREATMENT USED: _____
MOST EFFECTIVE TREATMENT: _____

TRIGGERS:
DIET 24 HOURS BEFORE MIGRAINE:
 - FOOD: _____
 - SNACKS: _____
 - ALCOHOL: _____
 - CAFFEINE: _____
 - WATER: _____
 - OTHER: _____

ODOURS: _____
STRESS: _____
CHANGES IN ROUTINE: _____
SLEEP PATTERN BEFORE MIGRAINE: _____
HORMONAL CHANGES (I.E. PERIOD): _____

POSSIBLE TRIGGERS FROM ABOVE INFORMATION: _____
NOTES: _____
_____
_____

DATE: _____

SEVERITY SCALE: 1 2 3 4 5 6 7 8 9 10

SYMPTOMS:
LIGHT SENSITIVITY: _   NAUSEA: _
SICKNESS: _   DIZZINESS: _
OTHER:_____

DURATION: _____

MEDICATION BEFORE MIGRAINE: _____
MEDICATION DURING MIGRAINE: _____
TREATMENT USED: _____
MOST EFFECTIVE TREATMENT: _____

TRIGGERS:
DIET 24 HOURS BEFORE MIGRAINE:
- FOOD: _____
- SNACKS: _____
- ALCOHOL: _____
- CAFFEINE: _____
- WATER: _____
- OTHER: _____

ODOURS: _____
STRESS: _____
CHANGES IN ROUTINE: _____
SLEEP PATTERN BEFORE MIGRAINE: _____
HORMONAL CHANGES (I.E. PERIOD): _____

POSSIBLE TRIGGERS FROM ABOVE INFORMATION: _____
NOTES: _____
_____
_____

DATE: _____

SEVERITY SCALE: 1 2 3 4 5 6 7 8 9 10

SYMPTOMS:
LIGHT SENSITIVITY: _   NAUSEA: _
SICKNESS: _   DIZZINESS: _
OTHER:_____

DURATION: _____

MEDICATION BEFORE MIGRAINE: _____
MEDICATION DURING MIGRAINE: _____
TREATMENT USED: _____
MOST EFFECTIVE TREATMENT: _____

TRIGGERS:
DIET 24 HOURS BEFORE MIGRAINE:
- FOOD: _____
- SNACKS: _____
- ALCOHOL: _____
- CAFFEINE: _____
- WATER: _____
- OTHER: _____

ODOURS: _____
STRESS: _____
CHANGES IN ROUTINE: _____
SLEEP PATTERN BEFORE MIGRAINE: _____
HORMONAL CHANGES (I.E. PERIOD): _____

POSSIBLE TRIGGERS FROM ABOVE INFORMATION: _____
NOTES: _____
_____
_____

DATE: _____

SEVERITY SCALE: 1 2 3 4 5 6 7 8 9 10

SYMPTOMS:
LIGHT SENSITIVITY: _   NAUSEA: _
SICKNESS: _   DIZZINESS: _
OTHER:_____

DURATION: _____

MEDICATION BEFORE MIGRAINE: _____
MEDICATION DURING MIGRAINE: _____
TREATMENT USED: _____
MOST EFFECTIVE TREATMENT: _____

TRIGGERS:
DIET 24 HOURS BEFORE MIGRAINE:
- FOOD: _____
- SNACKS: _____
- ALCOHOL: _____
- CAFFEINE: _____
- WATER: _____
- OTHER: _____

ODOURS: _____
STRESS: _____
CHANGES IN ROUTINE: _____
SLEEP PATTERN BEFORE MIGRAINE: _____
HORMONAL CHANGES (I.E. PERIOD): _____

POSSIBLE TRIGGERS FROM ABOVE INFORMATION: _____
NOTES: _____
_____
_____

DATE: _____

SEVERITY SCALE: 1 2 3 4 5 6 7 8 9 10

SYMPTOMS:
LIGHT SENSITIVITY: _   NAUSEA: _
SICKNESS: _   DIZZINESS: _
OTHER:_____

DURATION: _____

MEDICATION BEFORE MIGRAINE: _____
MEDICATION DURING MIGRAINE: _____
TREATMENT USED: _____
MOST EFFECTIVE TREATMENT: _____

TRIGGERS:
DIET 24 HOURS BEFORE MIGRAINE:
 - FOOD: _____
 - SNACKS: _____
 - ALCOHOL: _____
 - CAFFEINE: _____
 - WATER: _____
 - OTHER: _____

ODOURS: _____
STRESS: _____
CHANGES IN ROUTINE: _____
SLEEP PATTERN BEFORE MIGRAINE: _____
HORMONAL CHANGES (I.E. PERIOD): _____

POSSIBLE TRIGGERS FROM ABOVE INFORMATION: _____
NOTES: _____
_____
_____

DATE: _____

SEVERITY SCALE: 1 2 3 4 5 6 7 8 9 10

SYMPTOMS:
LIGHT SENSITIVITY: _   NAUSEA: _
SICKNESS: _   DIZZINESS: _
OTHER:_____

DURATION: _____

MEDICATION BEFORE MIGRAINE: _____
MEDICATION DURING MIGRAINE: _____
TREATMENT USED: _____
MOST EFFECTIVE TREATMENT: _____

TRIGGERS:
DIET 24 HOURS BEFORE MIGRAINE:
- FOOD: _____
- SNACKS: _____
- ALCOHOL: _____
- CAFFEINE: _____
- WATER: _____
- OTHER: _____

ODOURS: _____
STRESS: _____
CHANGES IN ROUTINE: _____
SLEEP PATTERN BEFORE MIGRAINE: _____
HORMONAL CHANGES (I.E. PERIOD): _____

POSSIBLE TRIGGERS FROM ABOVE INFORMATION: _____
NOTES: _____
_____
_____

DATE: _____

SEVERITY SCALE: 1 2 3 4 5 6 7 8 9 10

SYMPTOMS:
LIGHT SENSITIVITY: _   NAUSEA: _
SICKNESS: _   DIZZINESS: _
OTHER:_____

DURATION: _____

MEDICATION BEFORE MIGRAINE: _____
MEDICATION DURING MIGRAINE: _____
TREATMENT USED: _____
MOST EFFECTIVE TREATMENT: _____

TRIGGERS:
DIET 24 HOURS BEFORE MIGRAINE:
- FOOD: _____
- SNACKS: _____
- ALCOHOL: _____
- CAFFEINE: _____
- WATER: _____
- OTHER: _____

ODOURS: _____
STRESS: _____
CHANGES IN ROUTINE: _____
SLEEP PATTERN BEFORE MIGRAINE: _____
HORMONAL CHANGES (I.E. PERIOD): _____

POSSIBLE TRIGGERS FROM ABOVE INFORMATION: _____
NOTES: _____
_____
_____

DATE: _____

SEVERITY SCALE: 1 2 3 4 5 6 7 8 9 10

SYMPTOMS:
LIGHT SENSITIVITY: _   NAUSEA: _
SICKNESS: _   DIZZINESS: _
OTHER:_____

DURATION: _____

MEDICATION BEFORE MIGRAINE: _____
MEDICATION DURING MIGRAINE: _____
TREATMENT USED: _____
MOST EFFECTIVE TREATMENT: _____

TRIGGERS:
DIET 24 HOURS BEFORE MIGRAINE:
- FOOD: _____
- SNACKS: _____
- ALCOHOL: _____
- CAFFEINE: _____
- WATER: _____
- OTHER: _____

ODOURS: _____
STRESS: _____
CHANGES IN ROUTINE: _____
SLEEP PATTERN BEFORE MIGRAINE: _____
HORMONAL CHANGES (I.E. PERIOD): _____

POSSIBLE TRIGGERS FROM ABOVE INFORMATION: _____
NOTES: _____
_____
_____

DATE: _____

SEVERITY SCALE: 1 2 3 4 5 6 7 8 9 10

SYMPTOMS:
LIGHT SENSITIVITY: _   NAUSEA: _
SICKNESS: _   DIZZINESS: _
OTHER:_____

DURATION: _____

MEDICATION BEFORE MIGRAINE: _____
MEDICATION DURING MIGRAINE: _____
TREATMENT USED: _____
MOST EFFECTIVE TREATMENT: _____

TRIGGERS:
DIET 24 HOURS BEFORE MIGRAINE:
- FOOD: _____
- SNACKS: _____
- ALCOHOL: _____
- CAFFEINE: _____
- WATER: _____
- OTHER: _____

ODOURS: _____
STRESS: _____
CHANGES IN ROUTINE: _____
SLEEP PATTERN BEFORE MIGRAINE: _____
HORMONAL CHANGES (I.E. PERIOD): _____

POSSIBLE TRIGGERS FROM ABOVE INFORMATION: _____
NOTES: _____
_____
_____

DATE: _____

SEVERITY SCALE: 1 2 3 4 5 6 7 8 9 10

SYMPTOMS:
LIGHT SENSITIVITY: _   NAUSEA: _
SICKNESS: _   DIZZINESS: _
OTHER:_____

DURATION: _____

MEDICATION BEFORE MIGRAINE: _____
MEDICATION DURING MIGRAINE: _____
TREATMENT USED: _____
MOST EFFECTIVE TREATMENT: _____

TRIGGERS:
DIET 24 HOURS BEFORE MIGRAINE:
- FOOD: _____
- SNACKS: _____
- ALCOHOL: _____
- CAFFEINE: _____
- WATER: _____
- OTHER: _____

ODOURS: _____
STRESS: _____
CHANGES IN ROUTINE: _____
SLEEP PATTERN BEFORE MIGRAINE: _____
HORMONAL CHANGES (I.E. PERIOD): _____

POSSIBLE TRIGGERS FROM ABOVE INFORMATION: _____
NOTES: _____
_____
_____

DATE: _____

SEVERITY SCALE: 1 2 3 4 5 6 7 8 9 10

SYMPTOMS:
LIGHT SENSITIVITY: _   NAUSEA: _
SICKNESS: _   DIZZINESS: _
OTHER:_____

DURATION: _____

MEDICATION BEFORE MIGRAINE: _____
MEDICATION DURING MIGRAINE: _____
TREATMENT USED: _____
MOST EFFECTIVE TREATMENT: _____

TRIGGERS:
DIET 24 HOURS BEFORE MIGRAINE:
 - FOOD: _____
 - SNACKS: _____
 - ALCOHOL: _____
 - CAFFEINE: _____
 - WATER: _____
 - OTHER: _____

ODOURS: _____
STRESS: _____
CHANGES IN ROUTINE: _____
SLEEP PATTERN BEFORE MIGRAINE: _____
HORMONAL CHANGES (I.E. PERIOD): _____

POSSIBLE TRIGGERS FROM ABOVE INFORMATION: _____
NOTES: _____
_____
_____

DATE: _____

SEVERITY SCALE: 1 2 3 4 5 6 7 8 9 10

SYMPTOMS:
LIGHT SENSITIVITY: _   NAUSEA: _
SICKNESS: _   DIZZINESS: _
OTHER:_____

DURATION: _____

MEDICATION BEFORE MIGRAINE: _____
MEDICATION DURING MIGRAINE: _____
TREATMENT USED: _____
MOST EFFECTIVE TREATMENT: _____

TRIGGERS:
DIET 24 HOURS BEFORE MIGRAINE:
- FOOD: _____
- SNACKS: _____
- ALCOHOL: _____
- CAFFEINE: _____
- WATER: _____
- OTHER: _____

ODOURS: _____
STRESS: _____
CHANGES IN ROUTINE: _____
SLEEP PATTERN BEFORE MIGRAINE: _____
HORMONAL CHANGES (I.E. PERIOD): _____

POSSIBLE TRIGGERS FROM ABOVE INFORMATION: _____
NOTES: _____
_____
_____

DATE: _____

SEVERITY SCALE: 1 2 3 4 5 6 7 8 9 10

SYMPTOMS:
LIGHT SENSITIVITY: _   NAUSEA: _
SICKNESS: _   DIZZINESS: _
OTHER:_____

DURATION: _____

MEDICATION BEFORE MIGRAINE: _____
MEDICATION DURING MIGRAINE: _____
TREATMENT USED: _____
MOST EFFECTIVE TREATMENT: _____

TRIGGERS:
DIET 24 HOURS BEFORE MIGRAINE:
- FOOD: _____
- SNACKS: _____
- ALCOHOL: _____
- CAFFEINE: _____
- WATER: _____
- OTHER: _____

ODOURS: _____
STRESS: _____
CHANGES IN ROUTINE: _____
SLEEP PATTERN BEFORE MIGRAINE: _____
HORMONAL CHANGES (I.E. PERIOD): _____

POSSIBLE TRIGGERS FROM ABOVE INFORMATION: _____
NOTES: _____
_____
_____

DATE: _____

SEVERITY SCALE: 1 2 3 4 5 6 7 8 9 10

SYMPTOMS:
LIGHT SENSITIVITY: _   NAUSEA: _
SICKNESS: _   DIZZINESS: _
OTHER:_____

DURATION: _____

MEDICATION BEFORE MIGRAINE: _____
MEDICATION DURING MIGRAINE: _____
TREATMENT USED: _____
MOST EFFECTIVE TREATMENT: _____

TRIGGERS:
DIET 24 HOURS BEFORE MIGRAINE:
- FOOD: _____
- SNACKS: _____
- ALCOHOL: _____
- CAFFEINE: _____
- WATER: _____
- OTHER: _____

ODOURS: _____
STRESS: _____
CHANGES IN ROUTINE: _____
SLEEP PATTERN BEFORE MIGRAINE: _____
HORMONAL CHANGES (I.E. PERIOD): _____

POSSIBLE TRIGGERS FROM ABOVE INFORMATION: _____
NOTES: _____
_____
_____

DATE: _____

SEVERITY SCALE: 1 2 3 4 5 6 7 8 9 10

SYMPTOMS:
LIGHT SENSITIVITY: _   NAUSEA: _
SICKNESS: _   DIZZINESS: _
OTHER:_____

DURATION: _____

MEDICATION BEFORE MIGRAINE: _____
MEDICATION DURING MIGRAINE: _____
TREATMENT USED: _____
MOST EFFECTIVE TREATMENT: _____

TRIGGERS:
DIET 24 HOURS BEFORE MIGRAINE:
- FOOD: _____
- SNACKS: _____
- ALCOHOL: _____
- CAFFEINE: _____
- WATER: _____
- OTHER: _____

ODOURS: _____
STRESS: _____
CHANGES IN ROUTINE: _____
SLEEP PATTERN BEFORE MIGRAINE: _____
HORMONAL CHANGES (I.E. PERIOD): _____

POSSIBLE TRIGGERS FROM ABOVE INFORMATION: _____
NOTES: _____
_____
_____

DATE: _____

SEVERITY SCALE: 1 2 3 4 5 6 7 8 9 10

SYMPTOMS:
LIGHT SENSITIVITY: _   NAUSEA: _
SICKNESS: _   DIZZINESS: _
OTHER:_____

DURATION: _____

MEDICATION BEFORE MIGRAINE: _____
MEDICATION DURING MIGRAINE: _____
TREATMENT USED: _____
MOST EFFECTIVE TREATMENT: _____

TRIGGERS:
DIET 24 HOURS BEFORE MIGRAINE:
- FOOD: _____
- SNACKS: _____
- ALCOHOL: _____
- CAFFEINE: _____
- WATER: _____
- OTHER: _____

ODOURS: _____
STRESS: _____
CHANGES IN ROUTINE: _____
SLEEP PATTERN BEFORE MIGRAINE: _____
HORMONAL CHANGES (I.E. PERIOD): _____

POSSIBLE TRIGGERS FROM ABOVE INFORMATION: _____
NOTES: _____
_____
_____

DATE: _____

SEVERITY SCALE: 1 2 3 4 5 6 7 8 9 10

SYMPTOMS:
LIGHT SENSITIVITY: _   NAUSEA: _
SICKNESS: _   DIZZINESS: _
OTHER:_____

DURATION: _____

MEDICATION BEFORE MIGRAINE: _____
MEDICATION DURING MIGRAINE: _____
TREATMENT USED: _____
MOST EFFECTIVE TREATMENT: _____

TRIGGERS:
DIET 24 HOURS BEFORE MIGRAINE:
 - FOOD: _____
 - SNACKS: _____
 - ALCOHOL: _____
 - CAFFEINE: _____
 - WATER: _____
 - OTHER: _____

ODOURS: _____
STRESS: _____
CHANGES IN ROUTINE: _____
SLEEP PATTERN BEFORE MIGRAINE: _____
HORMONAL CHANGES (I.E. PERIOD): _____

POSSIBLE TRIGGERS FROM ABOVE INFORMATION: _____
NOTES: _____
_____
_____

DATE: _____

SEVERITY SCALE: 1 2 3 4 5 6 7 8 9 10

SYMPTOMS:
LIGHT SENSITIVITY: _   NAUSEA: _
SICKNESS: _   DIZZINESS: _
OTHER:_____

DURATION: _____

MEDICATION BEFORE MIGRAINE: _____
MEDICATION DURING MIGRAINE: _____
TREATMENT USED: _____
MOST EFFECTIVE TREATMENT: _____

TRIGGERS:
DIET 24 HOURS BEFORE MIGRAINE:
- FOOD: _____
- SNACKS: _____
- ALCOHOL: _____
- CAFFEINE: _____
- WATER: _____
- OTHER: _____

ODOURS: _____
STRESS: _____
CHANGES IN ROUTINE: _____
SLEEP PATTERN BEFORE MIGRAINE: _____
HORMONAL CHANGES (I.E. PERIOD): _____

POSSIBLE TRIGGERS FROM ABOVE INFORMATION: _____
NOTES: _____
_____
_____

DATE: _____

SEVERITY SCALE: 1 2 3 4 5 6 7 8 9 10

SYMPTOMS:
LIGHT SENSITIVITY: _   NAUSEA: _
SICKNESS: _   DIZZINESS: _
OTHER:_____

DURATION: _____

MEDICATION BEFORE MIGRAINE: _____
MEDICATION DURING MIGRAINE: _____
TREATMENT USED: _____
MOST EFFECTIVE TREATMENT: _____

TRIGGERS:
DIET 24 HOURS BEFORE MIGRAINE:
- FOOD: _____
- SNACKS: _____
- ALCOHOL: _____
- CAFFEINE: _____
- WATER: _____
- OTHER: _____

ODOURS: _____
STRESS: _____
CHANGES IN ROUTINE: _____
SLEEP PATTERN BEFORE MIGRAINE: _____
HORMONAL CHANGES (I.E. PERIOD): _____

POSSIBLE TRIGGERS FROM ABOVE INFORMATION: _____
NOTES: _____
_____
_____

DATE: _____

SEVERITY SCALE: 1 2 3 4 5 6 7 8 9 10

SYMPTOMS:
LIGHT SENSITIVITY: _   NAUSEA: _
SICKNESS: _   DIZZINESS: _
OTHER:_____

DURATION: _____

MEDICATION BEFORE MIGRAINE: _____
MEDICATION DURING MIGRAINE: _____
TREATMENT USED: _____
MOST EFFECTIVE TREATMENT: _____

TRIGGERS:
DIET 24 HOURS BEFORE MIGRAINE:
- FOOD: _____
- SNACKS: _____
- ALCOHOL: _____
- CAFFEINE: _____
- WATER: _____
- OTHER: _____

ODOURS: _____
STRESS: _____
CHANGES IN ROUTINE: _____
SLEEP PATTERN BEFORE MIGRAINE: _____
HORMONAL CHANGES (I.E. PERIOD): _____

POSSIBLE TRIGGERS FROM ABOVE INFORMATION: _____
NOTES: _____
_____
_____

DATE: _____

SEVERITY SCALE: 1 2 3 4 5 6 7 8 9 10

SYMPTOMS:
LIGHT SENSITIVITY: _   NAUSEA: _
SICKNESS: _   DIZZINESS: _
OTHER:_____

DURATION: _____

MEDICATION BEFORE MIGRAINE: _____
MEDICATION DURING MIGRAINE: _____
TREATMENT USED: _____
MOST EFFECTIVE TREATMENT: _____

TRIGGERS:
DIET 24 HOURS BEFORE MIGRAINE:
- FOOD: _____
- SNACKS: _____
- ALCOHOL: _____
- CAFFEINE: _____
- WATER: _____
- OTHER: _____

ODOURS: _____
STRESS: _____
CHANGES IN ROUTINE: _____
SLEEP PATTERN BEFORE MIGRAINE: _____
HORMONAL CHANGES (I.E. PERIOD): _____

POSSIBLE TRIGGERS FROM ABOVE INFORMATION: _____
NOTES: _____
_____
_____

DATE: _____

SEVERITY SCALE: 1 2 3 4 5 6 7 8 9 10

SYMPTOMS:
LIGHT SENSITIVITY: _   NAUSEA: _
SICKNESS: _   DIZZINESS: _
OTHER:_____

DURATION: _____

MEDICATION BEFORE MIGRAINE: _____
MEDICATION DURING MIGRAINE: _____
TREATMENT USED: _____
MOST EFFECTIVE TREATMENT: _____

TRIGGERS:
DIET 24 HOURS BEFORE MIGRAINE:
- FOOD: _____
- SNACKS: _____
- ALCOHOL: _____
- CAFFEINE: _____
- WATER: _____
- OTHER: _____

ODOURS: _____
STRESS: _____
CHANGES IN ROUTINE: _____
SLEEP PATTERN BEFORE MIGRAINE: _____
HORMONAL CHANGES (I.E. PERIOD): _____

POSSIBLE TRIGGERS FROM ABOVE INFORMATION: _____
NOTES: _____
_____
_____

DATE: _____

SEVERITY SCALE: 1 2 3 4 5 6 7 8 9 10

SYMPTOMS:
LIGHT SENSITIVITY: _   NAUSEA: _
SICKNESS: _   DIZZINESS: _
OTHER:_____

DURATION: _____

MEDICATION BEFORE MIGRAINE: _____
MEDICATION DURING MIGRAINE: _____
TREATMENT USED: _____
MOST EFFECTIVE TREATMENT: _____

TRIGGERS:
DIET 24 HOURS BEFORE MIGRAINE:
- FOOD: _____
- SNACKS: _____
- ALCOHOL: _____
- CAFFEINE: _____
- WATER: _____
- OTHER: _____

ODOURS: _____
STRESS: _____
CHANGES IN ROUTINE: _____
SLEEP PATTERN BEFORE MIGRAINE: _____
HORMONAL CHANGES (I.E. PERIOD): _____

POSSIBLE TRIGGERS FROM ABOVE INFORMATION: _____
NOTES: _____
_____
_____

DATE: _____

SEVERITY SCALE: 1 2 3 4 5 6 7 8 9 10

SYMPTOMS:
LIGHT SENSITIVITY: _   NAUSEA: _
SICKNESS: _   DIZZINESS: _
OTHER:_____

DURATION: _____

MEDICATION BEFORE MIGRAINE: _____
MEDICATION DURING MIGRAINE: _____
TREATMENT USED: _____
MOST EFFECTIVE TREATMENT: _____

TRIGGERS:
DIET 24 HOURS BEFORE MIGRAINE:
- FOOD: _____
- SNACKS: _____
- ALCOHOL: _____
- CAFFEINE: _____
- WATER: _____
- OTHER: _____

ODOURS: _____
STRESS: _____
CHANGES IN ROUTINE: _____
SLEEP PATTERN BEFORE MIGRAINE: _____
HORMONAL CHANGES (I.E. PERIOD): _____

POSSIBLE TRIGGERS FROM ABOVE INFORMATION: _____
NOTES: _____
_____
_____

DATE: _____

SEVERITY SCALE: 1 2 3 4 5 6 7 8 9 10

SYMPTOMS:
LIGHT SENSITIVITY: _   NAUSEA: _
SICKNESS: _   DIZZINESS: _
OTHER:_____

DURATION: _____

MEDICATION BEFORE MIGRAINE: _____
MEDICATION DURING MIGRAINE: _____
TREATMENT USED: _____
MOST EFFECTIVE TREATMENT: _____

TRIGGERS:
DIET 24 HOURS BEFORE MIGRAINE:
- FOOD: _____
- SNACKS: _____
- ALCOHOL: _____
- CAFFEINE: _____
- WATER: _____
- OTHER: _____

ODOURS: _____
STRESS: _____
CHANGES IN ROUTINE: _____
SLEEP PATTERN BEFORE MIGRAINE: _____
HORMONAL CHANGES (I.E. PERIOD): _____

POSSIBLE TRIGGERS FROM ABOVE INFORMATION: _____
NOTES: _____
_____
_____

DATE: _____

SEVERITY SCALE: 1 2 3 4 5 6 7 8 9 10

SYMPTOMS:
LIGHT SENSITIVITY: _   NAUSEA: _
SICKNESS: _   DIZZINESS: _
OTHER:_____

DURATION: _____

MEDICATION BEFORE MIGRAINE: _____
MEDICATION DURING MIGRAINE: _____
TREATMENT USED: _____
MOST EFFECTIVE TREATMENT: _____

TRIGGERS:
DIET 24 HOURS BEFORE MIGRAINE:
- FOOD: _____
- SNACKS: _____
- ALCOHOL: _____
- CAFFEINE: _____
- WATER: _____
- OTHER: _____

ODOURS: _____
STRESS: _____
CHANGES IN ROUTINE: _____
SLEEP PATTERN BEFORE MIGRAINE: _____
HORMONAL CHANGES (I.E. PERIOD): _____

POSSIBLE TRIGGERS FROM ABOVE INFORMATION: _____
NOTES: _____
_____
_____

DATE: _____

SEVERITY SCALE: 1 2 3 4 5 6 7 8 9 10

SYMPTOMS:
LIGHT SENSITIVITY: _   NAUSEA: _
SICKNESS: _   DIZZINESS: _
OTHER:_____

DURATION: _____

MEDICATION BEFORE MIGRAINE: _____
MEDICATION DURING MIGRAINE: _____
TREATMENT USED: _____
MOST EFFECTIVE TREATMENT: _____

TRIGGERS:
DIET 24 HOURS BEFORE MIGRAINE:
- FOOD: _____
- SNACKS: _____
- ALCOHOL: _____
- CAFFEINE: _____
- WATER: _____
- OTHER: _____

ODOURS: _____
STRESS: _____
CHANGES IN ROUTINE: _____
SLEEP PATTERN BEFORE MIGRAINE: _____
HORMONAL CHANGES (I.E. PERIOD): _____

POSSIBLE TRIGGERS FROM ABOVE INFORMATION: _____
NOTES: _____
_____
_____

DATE: _____

SEVERITY SCALE: 1 2 3 4 5 6 7 8 9 10

SYMPTOMS:
LIGHT SENSITIVITY: _   NAUSEA: _
SICKNESS: _   DIZZINESS: _
OTHER:_____

DURATION: _____

MEDICATION BEFORE MIGRAINE: _____
MEDICATION DURING MIGRAINE: _____
TREATMENT USED: _____
MOST EFFECTIVE TREATMENT: _____

TRIGGERS:
DIET 24 HOURS BEFORE MIGRAINE:
- FOOD: _____
- SNACKS: _____
- ALCOHOL: _____
- CAFFEINE: _____
- WATER: _____
- OTHER: _____

ODOURS: _____
STRESS: _____
CHANGES IN ROUTINE: _____
SLEEP PATTERN BEFORE MIGRAINE: _____
HORMONAL CHANGES (I.E. PERIOD): _____

POSSIBLE TRIGGERS FROM ABOVE INFORMATION: _____
NOTES: _____
_____
_____

DATE: _____

SEVERITY SCALE: 1 2 3 4 5 6 7 8 9 10

SYMPTOMS:
LIGHT SENSITIVITY: _   NAUSEA: _
SICKNESS: _   DIZZINESS: _
OTHER:_____

DURATION: _____

MEDICATION BEFORE MIGRAINE: _____
MEDICATION DURING MIGRAINE: _____
TREATMENT USED: _____
MOST EFFECTIVE TREATMENT: _____

TRIGGERS:
DIET 24 HOURS BEFORE MIGRAINE:
- FOOD: _____
- SNACKS: _____
- ALCOHOL: _____
- CAFFEINE: _____
- WATER: _____
- OTHER: _____

ODOURS: _____
STRESS: _____
CHANGES IN ROUTINE: _____
SLEEP PATTERN BEFORE MIGRAINE: _____
HORMONAL CHANGES (I.E. PERIOD): _____

POSSIBLE TRIGGERS FROM ABOVE INFORMATION: _____
NOTES: _____
_____
_____

DATE: _____

SEVERITY SCALE: 1 2 3 4 5 6 7 8 9 10

SYMPTOMS:

LIGHT SENSITIVITY: _   NAUSEA: _

SICKNESS: _   DIZZINESS: _

OTHER:_____

DURATION: _____

MEDICATION BEFORE MIGRAINE: _____

MEDICATION DURING MIGRAINE: _____

TREATMENT USED: _____

MOST EFFECTIVE TREATMENT: _____

TRIGGERS:

DIET 24 HOURS BEFORE MIGRAINE:

- FOOD: _____

- SNACKS: _____

- ALCOHOL: _____

- CAFFEINE: _____

- WATER: _____

- OTHER: _____

ODOURS: _____

STRESS: _____

CHANGES IN ROUTINE: _____

SLEEP PATTERN BEFORE MIGRAINE: _____

HORMONAL CHANGES (I.E. PERIOD): _____

POSSIBLE TRIGGERS FROM ABOVE INFORMATION: _____

NOTES: _____

_____

_____

DATE: _____

SEVERITY SCALE: 1 2 3 4 5 6 7 8 9 10

SYMPTOMS:
LIGHT SENSITIVITY: _   NAUSEA: _
SICKNESS: _   DIZZINESS: _
OTHER:_____

DURATION: _____

MEDICATION BEFORE MIGRAINE: _____
MEDICATION DURING MIGRAINE: _____
TREATMENT USED: _____
MOST EFFECTIVE TREATMENT: _____

TRIGGERS:
DIET 24 HOURS BEFORE MIGRAINE:
- FOOD: _____
- SNACKS: _____
- ALCOHOL: _____
- CAFFEINE: _____
- WATER: _____
- OTHER: _____

ODOURS: _____
STRESS: _____
CHANGES IN ROUTINE: _____
SLEEP PATTERN BEFORE MIGRAINE: _____
HORMONAL CHANGES (I.E. PERIOD): _____

POSSIBLE TRIGGERS FROM ABOVE INFORMATION: _____
NOTES: _____
_____
_____

DATE: _____

SEVERITY SCALE: 1 2 3 4 5 6 7 8 9 10

SYMPTOMS:
LIGHT SENSITIVITY: _   NAUSEA: _
SICKNESS: _   DIZZINESS: _
OTHER:_____

DURATION: _____

MEDICATION BEFORE MIGRAINE: _____
MEDICATION DURING MIGRAINE: _____
TREATMENT USED: _____
MOST EFFECTIVE TREATMENT: _____

TRIGGERS:
DIET 24 HOURS BEFORE MIGRAINE:
- FOOD: _____
- SNACKS: _____
- ALCOHOL: _____
- CAFFEINE: _____
- WATER: _____
- OTHER: _____

ODOURS: _____
STRESS: _____
CHANGES IN ROUTINE: _____
SLEEP PATTERN BEFORE MIGRAINE: _____
HORMONAL CHANGES (I.E. PERIOD): _____

POSSIBLE TRIGGERS FROM ABOVE INFORMATION: _____
NOTES: _____
_____
_____

DATE: _____

SEVERITY SCALE: 1 2 3 4 5 6 7 8 9 10

SYMPTOMS:
LIGHT SENSITIVITY: _   NAUSEA: _
SICKNESS: _   DIZZINESS: _
OTHER:_____

DURATION: _____

MEDICATION BEFORE MIGRAINE: _____
MEDICATION DURING MIGRAINE: _____
TREATMENT USED: _____
MOST EFFECTIVE TREATMENT: _____

TRIGGERS:
DIET 24 HOURS BEFORE MIGRAINE:
- FOOD: _____
- SNACKS: _____
- ALCOHOL: _____
- CAFFEINE: _____
- WATER: _____
- OTHER: _____

ODOURS: _____
STRESS: _____
CHANGES IN ROUTINE: _____
SLEEP PATTERN BEFORE MIGRAINE: _____
HORMONAL CHANGES (I.E. PERIOD): _____

POSSIBLE TRIGGERS FROM ABOVE INFORMATION: _____
NOTES: _____
_____
_____

DATE: _____

SEVERITY SCALE: 1 2 3 4 5 6 7 8 9 10

SYMPTOMS:
LIGHT SENSITIVITY: _   NAUSEA: _
SICKNESS: _   DIZZINESS: _
OTHER:_____

DURATION: _____

MEDICATION BEFORE MIGRAINE: _____
MEDICATION DURING MIGRAINE: _____
TREATMENT USED: _____
MOST EFFECTIVE TREATMENT: _____

TRIGGERS:
DIET 24 HOURS BEFORE MIGRAINE:
- FOOD: _____
- SNACKS: _____
- ALCOHOL: _____
- CAFFEINE: _____
- WATER: _____
- OTHER: _____

ODOURS: _____
STRESS: _____
CHANGES IN ROUTINE: _____
SLEEP PATTERN BEFORE MIGRAINE: _____
HORMONAL CHANGES (I.E. PERIOD): _____

POSSIBLE TRIGGERS FROM ABOVE INFORMATION: _____
NOTES: _____
_____
_____

DATE: _____

SEVERITY SCALE: 1   2   3   4   5   6   7   8   9   10

SYMPTOMS:
LIGHT SENSITIVITY: _   NAUSEA: _
SICKNESS: _   DIZZINESS: _
OTHER:_____

DURATION: _____

MEDICATION BEFORE MIGRAINE: _____
MEDICATION DURING MIGRAINE: _____
TREATMENT USED: _____
MOST EFFECTIVE TREATMENT: _____

TRIGGERS:
DIET 24 HOURS BEFORE MIGRAINE:
- FOOD: _____
- SNACKS: _____
- ALCOHOL: _____
- CAFFEINE: _____
- WATER: _____
- OTHER: _____

ODOURS: _____
STRESS: _____
CHANGES IN ROUTINE: _____
SLEEP PATTERN BEFORE MIGRAINE: _____
HORMONAL CHANGES (I.E. PERIOD): _____

POSSIBLE TRIGGERS FROM ABOVE INFORMATION: _____
NOTES: _____
_____
_____

DATE: _____

SEVERITY SCALE: 1 2 3 4 5 6 7 8 9 10

SYMPTOMS:
LIGHT SENSITIVITY: _   NAUSEA: _
SICKNESS: _   DIZZINESS: _
OTHER:_____

DURATION: _____

MEDICATION BEFORE MIGRAINE: _____
MEDICATION DURING MIGRAINE: _____
TREATMENT USED: _____
MOST EFFECTIVE TREATMENT: _____

TRIGGERS:
DIET 24 HOURS BEFORE MIGRAINE:
- FOOD: _____
- SNACKS: _____
- ALCOHOL: _____
- CAFFEINE: _____
- WATER: _____
- OTHER: _____

ODOURS: _____
STRESS: _____
CHANGES IN ROUTINE: _____
SLEEP PATTERN BEFORE MIGRAINE: _____
HORMONAL CHANGES (I.E. PERIOD): _____

POSSIBLE TRIGGERS FROM ABOVE INFORMATION: _____
NOTES: _____
_____
_____

DATE: _____

SEVERITY SCALE: 1 2 3 4 5 6 7 8 9 10

SYMPTOMS:
LIGHT SENSITIVITY: _   NAUSEA: _
SICKNESS: _   DIZZINESS: _
OTHER:_____

DURATION: _____

MEDICATION BEFORE MIGRAINE: _____
MEDICATION DURING MIGRAINE: _____
TREATMENT USED: _____
MOST EFFECTIVE TREATMENT: _____

TRIGGERS:
DIET 24 HOURS BEFORE MIGRAINE:
- FOOD: _____
- SNACKS: _____
- ALCOHOL: _____
- CAFFEINE: _____
- WATER: _____
- OTHER: _____

ODOURS: _____
STRESS: _____
CHANGES IN ROUTINE: _____
SLEEP PATTERN BEFORE MIGRAINE: _____
HORMONAL CHANGES (I.E. PERIOD): _____

POSSIBLE TRIGGERS FROM ABOVE INFORMATION: _____
NOTES: _____
_____
_____

DATE: _____

SEVERITY SCALE: 1 2 3 4 5 6 7 8 9 10

SYMPTOMS:
LIGHT SENSITIVITY: _   NAUSEA: _
SICKNESS: _   DIZZINESS: _
OTHER:_____

DURATION: _____

MEDICATION BEFORE MIGRAINE: _____
MEDICATION DURING MIGRAINE: _____
TREATMENT USED: _____
MOST EFFECTIVE TREATMENT: _____

TRIGGERS:
DIET 24 HOURS BEFORE MIGRAINE:
- FOOD: _____
- SNACKS: _____
- ALCOHOL: _____
- CAFFEINE: _____
- WATER: _____
- OTHER: _____

ODOURS: _____
STRESS: _____
CHANGES IN ROUTINE: _____
SLEEP PATTERN BEFORE MIGRAINE: _____
HORMONAL CHANGES (I.E. PERIOD): _____

POSSIBLE TRIGGERS FROM ABOVE INFORMATION: _____
NOTES: _____
_____
_____

DATE: _____

SEVERITY SCALE: 1 2 3 4 5 6 7 8 9 10

SYMPTOMS:
LIGHT SENSITIVITY: _   NAUSEA: _
SICKNESS: _   DIZZINESS: _
OTHER:_____

DURATION: _____

MEDICATION BEFORE MIGRAINE: _____
MEDICATION DURING MIGRAINE: _____
TREATMENT USED: _____
MOST EFFECTIVE TREATMENT: _____

TRIGGERS:
DIET 24 HOURS BEFORE MIGRAINE:
- FOOD: _____
- SNACKS: _____
- ALCOHOL: _____
- CAFFEINE: _____
- WATER: _____
- OTHER: _____

ODOURS: _____
STRESS: _____
CHANGES IN ROUTINE: _____
SLEEP PATTERN BEFORE MIGRAINE: _____
HORMONAL CHANGES (I.E. PERIOD): _____

POSSIBLE TRIGGERS FROM ABOVE INFORMATION: _____
NOTES: _____
_____
_____

DATE: _____

SEVERITY SCALE: 1 2 3 4 5 6 7 8 9 10

SYMPTOMS:
LIGHT SENSITIVITY: _   NAUSEA: _
SICKNESS: _   DIZZINESS: _
OTHER:_____

DURATION: _____

MEDICATION BEFORE MIGRAINE: _____
MEDICATION DURING MIGRAINE: _____
TREATMENT USED: _____
MOST EFFECTIVE TREATMENT: _____

TRIGGERS:
DIET 24 HOURS BEFORE MIGRAINE:
- FOOD: _____
- SNACKS: _____
- ALCOHOL: _____
- CAFFEINE: _____
- WATER: _____
- OTHER: _____

ODOURS: _____
STRESS: _____
CHANGES IN ROUTINE: _____
SLEEP PATTERN BEFORE MIGRAINE: _____
HORMONAL CHANGES (I.E. PERIOD): _____

POSSIBLE TRIGGERS FROM ABOVE INFORMATION: _____
NOTES: _____
_____
_____

DATE: _____

SEVERITY SCALE: 1 2 3 4 5 6 7 8 9 10

SYMPTOMS:
LIGHT SENSITIVITY: _   NAUSEA: _
SICKNESS: _   DIZZINESS: _
OTHER:_____

DURATION: _____

MEDICATION BEFORE MIGRAINE: _____
MEDICATION DURING MIGRAINE: _____
TREATMENT USED: _____
MOST EFFECTIVE TREATMENT: _____

TRIGGERS:
DIET 24 HOURS BEFORE MIGRAINE:
- FOOD: _____
- SNACKS: _____
- ALCOHOL: _____
- CAFFEINE: _____
- WATER: _____
- OTHER: _____

ODOURS: _____
STRESS: _____
CHANGES IN ROUTINE: _____
SLEEP PATTERN BEFORE MIGRAINE: _____
HORMONAL CHANGES (I.E. PERIOD): _____

POSSIBLE TRIGGERS FROM ABOVE INFORMATION: _____
NOTES: _____
_____
_____

DATE: _____

SEVERITY SCALE: 1 2 3 4 5 6 7 8 9 10

SYMPTOMS:
LIGHT SENSITIVITY: _   NAUSEA: _
SICKNESS: _   DIZZINESS: _
OTHER:_____

DURATION: _____

MEDICATION BEFORE MIGRAINE: _____
MEDICATION DURING MIGRAINE: _____
TREATMENT USED: _____
MOST EFFECTIVE TREATMENT: _____

TRIGGERS:
DIET 24 HOURS BEFORE MIGRAINE:
- FOOD: _____
- SNACKS: _____
- ALCOHOL: _____
- CAFFEINE: _____
- WATER: _____
- OTHER: _____

ODOURS: _____
STRESS: _____
CHANGES IN ROUTINE: _____
SLEEP PATTERN BEFORE MIGRAINE: _____
HORMONAL CHANGES (I.E. PERIOD): _____

POSSIBLE TRIGGERS FROM ABOVE INFORMATION: _____
NOTES: _____
_____
_____

DATE: _____

SEVERITY SCALE: 1 2 3 4 5 6 7 8 9 10

SYMPTOMS:
LIGHT SENSITIVITY: _   NAUSEA: _
SICKNESS: _   DIZZINESS: _
OTHER:_____

DURATION: _____

MEDICATION BEFORE MIGRAINE: _____
MEDICATION DURING MIGRAINE: _____
TREATMENT USED: _____
MOST EFFECTIVE TREATMENT: _____

TRIGGERS:
DIET 24 HOURS BEFORE MIGRAINE:
 - FOOD: _____
 - SNACKS: _____
 - ALCOHOL: _____
 - CAFFEINE: _____
 - WATER: _____
 - OTHER: _____

ODOURS: _____
STRESS: _____
CHANGES IN ROUTINE: _____
SLEEP PATTERN BEFORE MIGRAINE: _____
HORMONAL CHANGES (I.E. PERIOD): _____

POSSIBLE TRIGGERS FROM ABOVE INFORMATION: _____
NOTES: _____
_____
_____

DATE: _____

SEVERITY SCALE: 1 2 3 4 5 6 7 8 9 10

SYMPTOMS:
LIGHT SENSITIVITY: _   NAUSEA: _
SICKNESS: _   DIZZINESS: _
OTHER:_____

DURATION: _____

MEDICATION BEFORE MIGRAINE: _____
MEDICATION DURING MIGRAINE: _____
TREATMENT USED: _____
MOST EFFECTIVE TREATMENT: _____

TRIGGERS:
DIET 24 HOURS BEFORE MIGRAINE:
- FOOD: _____
- SNACKS: _____
- ALCOHOL: _____
- CAFFEINE: _____
- WATER: _____
- OTHER: _____

ODOURS: _____
STRESS: _____
CHANGES IN ROUTINE: _____
SLEEP PATTERN BEFORE MIGRAINE: _____
HORMONAL CHANGES (I.E. PERIOD): _____

POSSIBLE TRIGGERS FROM ABOVE INFORMATION: _____
NOTES: _____
_____
_____

DATE: _____

SEVERITY SCALE: 1   2   3   4   5   6   7   8   9   10

SYMPTOMS:
LIGHT SENSITIVITY: _   NAUSEA: _
SICKNESS: _   DIZZINESS: _
OTHER:_____

DURATION: _____

MEDICATION BEFORE MIGRAINE: _____
MEDICATION DURING MIGRAINE: _____
TREATMENT USED: _____
MOST EFFECTIVE TREATMENT: _____

TRIGGERS:
DIET 24 HOURS BEFORE MIGRAINE:
- FOOD: _____
- SNACKS: _____
- ALCOHOL: _____
- CAFFEINE: _____
- WATER: _____
- OTHER: _____

ODOURS: _____
STRESS: _____
CHANGES IN ROUTINE: _____
SLEEP PATTERN BEFORE MIGRAINE: _____
HORMONAL CHANGES (I.E. PERIOD): _____

POSSIBLE TRIGGERS FROM ABOVE INFORMATION: _____
NOTES: _____
_____
_____

DATE: _____

SEVERITY SCALE: 1 2 3 4 5 6 7 8 9 10

SYMPTOMS:
LIGHT SENSITIVITY: _   NAUSEA: _
SICKNESS: _   DIZZINESS: _
OTHER:_____

DURATION: _____

MEDICATION BEFORE MIGRAINE: _____
MEDICATION DURING MIGRAINE: _____
TREATMENT USED: _____
MOST EFFECTIVE TREATMENT: _____

TRIGGERS:
DIET 24 HOURS BEFORE MIGRAINE:
- FOOD: _____
- SNACKS: _____
- ALCOHOL: _____
- CAFFEINE: _____
- WATER: _____
- OTHER: _____

ODOURS: _____
STRESS: _____
CHANGES IN ROUTINE: _____
SLEEP PATTERN BEFORE MIGRAINE: _____
HORMONAL CHANGES (I.E. PERIOD): _____

POSSIBLE TRIGGERS FROM ABOVE INFORMATION: _____
NOTES: _____
_____
_____

DATE: _____

SEVERITY SCALE: 1 2 3 4 5 6 7 8 9 10

SYMPTOMS:
LIGHT SENSITIVITY: _   NAUSEA: _
SICKNESS: _   DIZZINESS: _
OTHER:_____

DURATION: _____

MEDICATION BEFORE MIGRAINE: _____
MEDICATION DURING MIGRAINE: _____
TREATMENT USED: _____
MOST EFFECTIVE TREATMENT: _____

TRIGGERS:
DIET 24 HOURS BEFORE MIGRAINE:
 - FOOD: _____
 - SNACKS: _____
 - ALCOHOL: _____
 - CAFFEINE: _____
 - WATER: _____
 - OTHER: _____

ODOURS: _____
STRESS: _____
CHANGES IN ROUTINE: _____
SLEEP PATTERN BEFORE MIGRAINE: _____
HORMONAL CHANGES (I.E. PERIOD): _____

POSSIBLE TRIGGERS FROM ABOVE INFORMATION: _____
NOTES: _____
_____
_____

DATE: _____

SEVERITY SCALE: 1 2 3 4 5 6 7 8 9 10

SYMPTOMS:
LIGHT SENSITIVITY: _   NAUSEA: _
SICKNESS: _   DIZZINESS: _
OTHER:_____

DURATION: _____

MEDICATION BEFORE MIGRAINE: _____
MEDICATION DURING MIGRAINE: _____
TREATMENT USED: _____
MOST EFFECTIVE TREATMENT: _____

TRIGGERS:
DIET 24 HOURS BEFORE MIGRAINE:
- FOOD: _____
- SNACKS: _____
- ALCOHOL: _____
- CAFFEINE: _____
- WATER: _____
- OTHER: _____

ODOURS: _____
STRESS: _____
CHANGES IN ROUTINE: _____
SLEEP PATTERN BEFORE MIGRAINE: _____
HORMONAL CHANGES (I.E. PERIOD): _____

POSSIBLE TRIGGERS FROM ABOVE INFORMATION: _____
NOTES: _____
_____
_____

DATE: _____

SEVERITY SCALE: 1 2 3 4 5 6 7 8 9 10

SYMPTOMS:
LIGHT SENSITIVITY: _   NAUSEA: _
SICKNESS: _   DIZZINESS: _
OTHER:_____

DURATION: _____

MEDICATION BEFORE MIGRAINE: _____
MEDICATION DURING MIGRAINE: _____
TREATMENT USED: _____
MOST EFFECTIVE TREATMENT: _____

TRIGGERS:
DIET 24 HOURS BEFORE MIGRAINE:
- FOOD: _____
- SNACKS: _____
- ALCOHOL: _____
- CAFFEINE: _____
- WATER: _____
- OTHER: _____

ODOURS: _____
STRESS: _____
CHANGES IN ROUTINE: _____
SLEEP PATTERN BEFORE MIGRAINE: _____
HORMONAL CHANGES (I.E. PERIOD): _____

POSSIBLE TRIGGERS FROM ABOVE INFORMATION: _____
NOTES: _____
_____
_____

DATE: _____

SEVERITY SCALE: 1 2 3 4 5 6 7 8 9 10

SYMPTOMS:
LIGHT SENSITIVITY: _   NAUSEA: _
SICKNESS: _   DIZZINESS: _
OTHER:_____

DURATION: _____

MEDICATION BEFORE MIGRAINE: _____
MEDICATION DURING MIGRAINE: _____
TREATMENT USED: _____
MOST EFFECTIVE TREATMENT: _____

TRIGGERS:
DIET 24 HOURS BEFORE MIGRAINE:
- FOOD: _____
- SNACKS: _____
- ALCOHOL: _____
- CAFFEINE: _____
- WATER: _____
- OTHER: _____

ODOURS: _____
STRESS: _____
CHANGES IN ROUTINE: _____
SLEEP PATTERN BEFORE MIGRAINE: _____
HORMONAL CHANGES (I.E. PERIOD): _____

POSSIBLE TRIGGERS FROM ABOVE INFORMATION: _____
NOTES: _____
_____
_____

DATE: _____

SEVERITY SCALE: 1 2 3 4 5 6 7 8 9 10

SYMPTOMS:
LIGHT SENSITIVITY: _   NAUSEA: _
SICKNESS: _   DIZZINESS: _
OTHER:_____

DURATION: _____

MEDICATION BEFORE MIGRAINE: _____
MEDICATION DURING MIGRAINE: _____
TREATMENT USED: _____
MOST EFFECTIVE TREATMENT: _____

TRIGGERS:
DIET 24 HOURS BEFORE MIGRAINE:
- FOOD: _____
- SNACKS: _____
- ALCOHOL: _____
- CAFFEINE: _____
- WATER: _____
- OTHER: _____

ODOURS: _____
STRESS: _____
CHANGES IN ROUTINE: _____
SLEEP PATTERN BEFORE MIGRAINE: _____
HORMONAL CHANGES (I.E. PERIOD): _____

POSSIBLE TRIGGERS FROM ABOVE INFORMATION: _____
NOTES: _____
_____
_____

DATE: _____

SEVERITY SCALE: 1 2 3 4 5 6 7 8 9 10

SYMPTOMS:
LIGHT SENSITIVITY: _   NAUSEA: _
SICKNESS: _   DIZZINESS: _
OTHER:_____

DURATION: _____

MEDICATION BEFORE MIGRAINE: _____
MEDICATION DURING MIGRAINE: _____
TREATMENT USED: _____
MOST EFFECTIVE TREATMENT: _____

TRIGGERS:
DIET 24 HOURS BEFORE MIGRAINE:
- FOOD: _____
- SNACKS: _____
- ALCOHOL: _____
- CAFFEINE: _____
- WATER: _____
- OTHER: _____

ODOURS: _____
STRESS: _____
CHANGES IN ROUTINE: _____
SLEEP PATTERN BEFORE MIGRAINE: _____
HORMONAL CHANGES (I.E. PERIOD): _____

POSSIBLE TRIGGERS FROM ABOVE INFORMATION: _____
NOTES: _____
_____
_____

DATE: _____

SEVERITY SCALE: 1 2 3 4 5 6 7 8 9 10

SYMPTOMS:
LIGHT SENSITIVITY: _   NAUSEA: _
SICKNESS: _   DIZZINESS: _
OTHER:_____

DURATION: _____

MEDICATION BEFORE MIGRAINE: _____
MEDICATION DURING MIGRAINE: _____
TREATMENT USED: _____
MOST EFFECTIVE TREATMENT: _____

TRIGGERS:
DIET 24 HOURS BEFORE MIGRAINE:
– FOOD: _____
– SNACKS: _____
– ALCOHOL: _____
– CAFFEINE: _____
– WATER: _____
– OTHER: _____

ODOURS: _____
STRESS: _____
CHANGES IN ROUTINE: _____
SLEEP PATTERN BEFORE MIGRAINE: _____
HORMONAL CHANGES (I.E. PERIOD): _____

POSSIBLE TRIGGERS FROM ABOVE INFORMATION: _____
NOTES: _____
_____
_____

DATE: _____

SEVERITY SCALE: 1 2 3 4 5 6 7 8 9 10

SYMPTOMS:
LIGHT SENSITIVITY: _   NAUSEA: _
SICKNESS: _   DIZZINESS: _
OTHER:_____

DURATION: _____

MEDICATION BEFORE MIGRAINE: _____
MEDICATION DURING MIGRAINE: _____
TREATMENT USED: _____
MOST EFFECTIVE TREATMENT: _____

TRIGGERS:
DIET 24 HOURS BEFORE MIGRAINE:
- FOOD: _____
- SNACKS: _____
- ALCOHOL: _____
- CAFFEINE: _____
- WATER: _____
- OTHER: _____

ODOURS: _____
STRESS: _____
CHANGES IN ROUTINE: _____
SLEEP PATTERN BEFORE MIGRAINE: _____
HORMONAL CHANGES (I.E. PERIOD): _____

POSSIBLE TRIGGERS FROM ABOVE INFORMATION: _____
NOTES: _____
_____
_____

DATE: _____

SEVERITY SCALE: 1 2 3 4 5 6 7 8 9 10

SYMPTOMS:
LIGHT SENSITIVITY: _   NAUSEA: _
SICKNESS: _   DIZZINESS: _
OTHER:_____

DURATION: _____

MEDICATION BEFORE MIGRAINE: _____
MEDICATION DURING MIGRAINE: _____
TREATMENT USED: _____
MOST EFFECTIVE TREATMENT: _____

TRIGGERS:
DIET 24 HOURS BEFORE MIGRAINE:
- FOOD: _____
- SNACKS: _____
- ALCOHOL: _____
- CAFFEINE: _____
- WATER: _____
- OTHER: _____

ODOURS: _____
STRESS: _____
CHANGES IN ROUTINE: _____
SLEEP PATTERN BEFORE MIGRAINE: _____
HORMONAL CHANGES (I.E. PERIOD): _____

POSSIBLE TRIGGERS FROM ABOVE INFORMATION: _____
NOTES: _____
_____
_____

DATE: _____

SEVERITY SCALE: 1 2 3 4 5 6 7 8 9 10

SYMPTOMS:
LIGHT SENSITIVITY: _   NAUSEA: _
SICKNESS: _   DIZZINESS: _
OTHER:_____

DURATION: _____

MEDICATION BEFORE MIGRAINE: _____
MEDICATION DURING MIGRAINE: _____
TREATMENT USED: _____
MOST EFFECTIVE TREATMENT: _____

TRIGGERS:
DIET 24 HOURS BEFORE MIGRAINE:
- FOOD: _____
- SNACKS: _____
- ALCOHOL: _____
- CAFFEINE: _____
- WATER: _____
- OTHER: _____

ODOURS: _____
STRESS: _____
CHANGES IN ROUTINE: _____
SLEEP PATTERN BEFORE MIGRAINE: _____
HORMONAL CHANGES (I.E. PERIOD): _____

POSSIBLE TRIGGERS FROM ABOVE INFORMATION: _____
NOTES: _____
_____
_____

DATE: _____

SEVERITY SCALE: 1 2 3 4 5 6 7 8 9 10

SYMPTOMS:
LIGHT SENSITIVITY: _   NAUSEA: _
SICKNESS: _   DIZZINESS: _
OTHER:_____

DURATION: _____

MEDICATION BEFORE MIGRAINE: _____
MEDICATION DURING MIGRAINE: _____
TREATMENT USED: _____
MOST EFFECTIVE TREATMENT: _____

TRIGGERS:
DIET 24 HOURS BEFORE MIGRAINE:
- FOOD: _____
- SNACKS: _____
- ALCOHOL: _____
- CAFFEINE: _____
- WATER: _____
- OTHER: _____

ODOURS: _____
STRESS: _____
CHANGES IN ROUTINE: _____
SLEEP PATTERN BEFORE MIGRAINE: _____
HORMONAL CHANGES (I.E. PERIOD): _____

POSSIBLE TRIGGERS FROM ABOVE INFORMATION: _____
NOTES: _____
_____
_____

DATE: _____

SEVERITY SCALE: 1 2 3 4 5 6 7 8 9 10

SYMPTOMS:
LIGHT SENSITIVITY: _   NAUSEA: _
SICKNESS: _   DIZZINESS: _
OTHER:_____

DURATION: _____

MEDICATION BEFORE MIGRAINE: _____
MEDICATION DURING MIGRAINE: _____
TREATMENT USED: _____
MOST EFFECTIVE TREATMENT: _____

TRIGGERS:
DIET 24 HOURS BEFORE MIGRAINE:
- FOOD: _____
- SNACKS: _____
- ALCOHOL: _____
- CAFFEINE: _____
- WATER: _____
- OTHER: _____

ODOURS: _____
STRESS: _____
CHANGES IN ROUTINE: _____
SLEEP PATTERN BEFORE MIGRAINE: _____
HORMONAL CHANGES (I.E. PERIOD): _____

POSSIBLE TRIGGERS FROM ABOVE INFORMATION: _____
NOTES: _____
_____
_____

DATE: _____

SEVERITY SCALE: 1 2 3 4 5 6 7 8 9 10

SYMPTOMS:

LIGHT SENSITIVITY: _   NAUSEA: _

SICKNESS: _   DIZZINESS: _

OTHER:_____

DURATION: _____

MEDICATION BEFORE MIGRAINE: _____

MEDICATION DURING MIGRAINE: _____

TREATMENT USED: _____

MOST EFFECTIVE TREATMENT: _____

TRIGGERS:

DIET 24 HOURS BEFORE MIGRAINE:

- FOOD: _____
- SNACKS: _____
- ALCOHOL: _____
- CAFFEINE: _____
- WATER: _____
- OTHER: _____

ODOURS: _____

STRESS: _____

CHANGES IN ROUTINE: _____

SLEEP PATTERN BEFORE MIGRAINE: _____

HORMONAL CHANGES (I.E. PERIOD): _____

POSSIBLE TRIGGERS FROM ABOVE INFORMATION: _____

NOTES: _____

_____

_____

DATE: _____

SEVERITY SCALE: 1 2 3 4 5 6 7 8 9 10

SYMPTOMS:
LIGHT SENSITIVITY: _   NAUSEA: _
SICKNESS: _   DIZZINESS: _
OTHER:_____

DURATION: _____

MEDICATION BEFORE MIGRAINE: _____
MEDICATION DURING MIGRAINE: _____
TREATMENT USED: _____
MOST EFFECTIVE TREATMENT: _____

TRIGGERS:
DIET 24 HOURS BEFORE MIGRAINE:
- FOOD: _____
- SNACKS: _____
- ALCOHOL: _____
- CAFFEINE: _____
- WATER: _____
- OTHER: _____

ODOURS: _____
STRESS: _____
CHANGES IN ROUTINE: _____
SLEEP PATTERN BEFORE MIGRAINE: _____
HORMONAL CHANGES (I.E. PERIOD): _____

POSSIBLE TRIGGERS FROM ABOVE INFORMATION: _____
NOTES: _____
_____
_____

DATE: _____

SEVERITY SCALE: 1 2 3 4 5 6 7 8 9 10

SYMPTOMS:
LIGHT SENSITIVITY: _   NAUSEA: _
SICKNESS: _   DIZZINESS: _
OTHER:_____

DURATION: _____

MEDICATION BEFORE MIGRAINE: _____
MEDICATION DURING MIGRAINE: _____
TREATMENT USED: _____
MOST EFFECTIVE TREATMENT: _____

TRIGGERS:
DIET 24 HOURS BEFORE MIGRAINE:
- FOOD: _____
- SNACKS: _____
- ALCOHOL: _____
- CAFFEINE: _____
- WATER: _____
- OTHER: _____

ODOURS: _____
STRESS: _____
CHANGES IN ROUTINE: _____
SLEEP PATTERN BEFORE MIGRAINE: _____
HORMONAL CHANGES (I.E. PERIOD): _____

POSSIBLE TRIGGERS FROM ABOVE INFORMATION: _____
NOTES: _____
_____
_____

DATE: _____

SEVERITY SCALE: 1 2 3 4 5 6 7 8 9 10

SYMPTOMS:
LIGHT SENSITIVITY: _   NAUSEA: _
SICKNESS: _   DIZZINESS: _
OTHER:_____

DURATION: _____

MEDICATION BEFORE MIGRAINE: _____
MEDICATION DURING MIGRAINE: _____
TREATMENT USED: _____
MOST EFFECTIVE TREATMENT: _____

TRIGGERS:
DIET 24 HOURS BEFORE MIGRAINE:
- FOOD: _____
- SNACKS: _____
- ALCOHOL: _____
- CAFFEINE: _____
- WATER: _____
- OTHER: _____

ODOURS: _____
STRESS: _____
CHANGES IN ROUTINE: _____
SLEEP PATTERN BEFORE MIGRAINE: _____
HORMONAL CHANGES (I.E. PERIOD): _____

POSSIBLE TRIGGERS FROM ABOVE INFORMATION: _____
NOTES: _____
_____
_____

DATE: _____

SEVERITY SCALE: 1 2 3 4 5 6 7 8 9 10

SYMPTOMS:
LIGHT SENSITIVITY: _   NAUSEA: _
SICKNESS: _   DIZZINESS: _
OTHER:_____

DURATION: _____

MEDICATION BEFORE MIGRAINE: _____
MEDICATION DURING MIGRAINE: _____
TREATMENT USED: _____
MOST EFFECTIVE TREATMENT: _____

TRIGGERS:
DIET 24 HOURS BEFORE MIGRAINE:
- FOOD: _____
- SNACKS: _____
- ALCOHOL: _____
- CAFFEINE: _____
- WATER: _____
- OTHER: _____

ODOURS: _____
STRESS: _____
CHANGES IN ROUTINE: _____
SLEEP PATTERN BEFORE MIGRAINE: _____
HORMONAL CHANGES (I.E. PERIOD): _____

POSSIBLE TRIGGERS FROM ABOVE INFORMATION: _____
NOTES: _____
_____
_____

DATE: _____

SEVERITY SCALE: 1 2 3 4 5 6 7 8 9 10

SYMPTOMS:
LIGHT SENSITIVITY: _   NAUSEA: _
SICKNESS: _   DIZZINESS: _
OTHER:_____

DURATION: _____

MEDICATION BEFORE MIGRAINE: _____
MEDICATION DURING MIGRAINE: _____
TREATMENT USED: _____
MOST EFFECTIVE TREATMENT: _____

TRIGGERS:
DIET 24 HOURS BEFORE MIGRAINE:
- FOOD: _____
- SNACKS: _____
- ALCOHOL: _____
- CAFFEINE: _____
- WATER: _____
- OTHER: _____

ODOURS: _____
STRESS: _____
CHANGES IN ROUTINE: _____
SLEEP PATTERN BEFORE MIGRAINE: _____
HORMONAL CHANGES (I.E. PERIOD): _____

POSSIBLE TRIGGERS FROM ABOVE INFORMATION: _____
NOTES: _____
_____
_____

DATE: _____

SEVERITY SCALE: 1 2 3 4 5 6 7 8 9 10

SYMPTOMS:
LIGHT SENSITIVITY: _   NAUSEA: _
SICKNESS: _   DIZZINESS: _
OTHER:_____

DURATION: _____

MEDICATION BEFORE MIGRAINE: _____
MEDICATION DURING MIGRAINE: _____
TREATMENT USED: _____
MOST EFFECTIVE TREATMENT: _____

TRIGGERS:
DIET 24 HOURS BEFORE MIGRAINE:
 - FOOD: _____
 - SNACKS: _____
 - ALCOHOL: _____
 - CAFFEINE: _____
 - WATER: _____
 - OTHER: _____

ODOURS: _____
STRESS: _____
CHANGES IN ROUTINE: _____
SLEEP PATTERN BEFORE MIGRAINE: _____
HORMONAL CHANGES (I.E. PERIOD): _____

POSSIBLE TRIGGERS FROM ABOVE INFORMATION: _____
NOTES: _____
_____
_____

DATE: _____

SEVERITY SCALE: 1 2 3 4 5 6 7 8 9 10

SYMPTOMS:
LIGHT SENSITIVITY: _   NAUSEA: _
SICKNESS: _   DIZZINESS: _
OTHER:_____

DURATION: _____

MEDICATION BEFORE MIGRAINE: _____
MEDICATION DURING MIGRAINE: _____
TREATMENT USED: _____
MOST EFFECTIVE TREATMENT: _____

TRIGGERS:
DIET 24 HOURS BEFORE MIGRAINE:
- FOOD: _____
- SNACKS: _____
- ALCOHOL: _____
- CAFFEINE: _____
- WATER: _____
- OTHER: _____

ODOURS: _____
STRESS: _____
CHANGES IN ROUTINE: _____
SLEEP PATTERN BEFORE MIGRAINE: _____
HORMONAL CHANGES (I.E. PERIOD): _____

POSSIBLE TRIGGERS FROM ABOVE INFORMATION: _____
NOTES: _____
_____
_____

DATE: _____

SEVERITY SCALE: 1 2 3 4 5 6 7 8 9 10

SYMPTOMS:
LIGHT SENSITIVITY: _   NAUSEA: _
SICKNESS: _   DIZZINESS: _
OTHER:_____

DURATION: _____

MEDICATION BEFORE MIGRAINE: _____
MEDICATION DURING MIGRAINE: _____
TREATMENT USED: _____
MOST EFFECTIVE TREATMENT: _____

TRIGGERS:
DIET 24 HOURS BEFORE MIGRAINE:
- FOOD: _____
- SNACKS: _____
- ALCOHOL: _____
- CAFFEINE: _____
- WATER: _____
- OTHER: _____

ODOURS: _____
STRESS: _____
CHANGES IN ROUTINE: _____
SLEEP PATTERN BEFORE MIGRAINE: _____
HORMONAL CHANGES (I.E. PERIOD): _____

POSSIBLE TRIGGERS FROM ABOVE INFORMATION: _____
NOTES: _____
_____
_____

DATE: _____

SEVERITY SCALE: 1 2 3 4 5 6 7 8 9 10

SYMPTOMS:
LIGHT SENSITIVITY: _   NAUSEA: _
SICKNESS: _   DIZZINESS: _
OTHER:_____

DURATION: _____

MEDICATION BEFORE MIGRAINE: _____
MEDICATION DURING MIGRAINE: _____
TREATMENT USED: _____
MOST EFFECTIVE TREATMENT: _____

TRIGGERS:
DIET 24 HOURS BEFORE MIGRAINE:
 - FOOD: _____
 - SNACKS: _____
 - ALCOHOL: _____
 - CAFFEINE: _____
 - WATER: _____
 - OTHER: _____

ODOURS: _____
STRESS: _____
CHANGES IN ROUTINE: _____
SLEEP PATTERN BEFORE MIGRAINE: _____
HORMONAL CHANGES (I.E. PERIOD): _____

POSSIBLE TRIGGERS FROM ABOVE INFORMATION: _____
NOTES: _____
_____
_____

DATE: _____

SEVERITY SCALE: 1 2 3 4 5 6 7 8 9 10

SYMPTOMS:
LIGHT SENSITIVITY: _   NAUSEA: _
SICKNESS: _   DIZZINESS: _
OTHER:_____

DURATION: _____

MEDICATION BEFORE MIGRAINE: _____
MEDICATION DURING MIGRAINE: _____
TREATMENT USED: _____
MOST EFFECTIVE TREATMENT: _____

TRIGGERS:
DIET 24 HOURS BEFORE MIGRAINE:
- FOOD: _____
- SNACKS: _____
- ALCOHOL: _____
- CAFFEINE: _____
- WATER: _____
- OTHER: _____

ODOURS: _____
STRESS: _____
CHANGES IN ROUTINE: _____
SLEEP PATTERN BEFORE MIGRAINE: _____
HORMONAL CHANGES (I.E. PERIOD): _____

POSSIBLE TRIGGERS FROM ABOVE INFORMATION: _____
NOTES: _____
_____
_____

DATE: _____

SEVERITY SCALE: 1 2 3 4 5 6 7 8 9 10

SYMPTOMS:
LIGHT SENSITIVITY: _   NAUSEA: _
SICKNESS: _   DIZZINESS: _
OTHER:_____

DURATION: _____

MEDICATION BEFORE MIGRAINE: _____
MEDICATION DURING MIGRAINE: _____
TREATMENT USED: _____
MOST EFFECTIVE TREATMENT: _____

TRIGGERS:
DIET 24 HOURS BEFORE MIGRAINE:
- FOOD: _____
- SNACKS: _____
- ALCOHOL: _____
- CAFFEINE: _____
- WATER: _____
- OTHER: _____

ODOURS: _____
STRESS: _____
CHANGES IN ROUTINE: _____
SLEEP PATTERN BEFORE MIGRAINE: _____
HORMONAL CHANGES (I.E. PERIOD): _____

POSSIBLE TRIGGERS FROM ABOVE INFORMATION: _____
NOTES: _____
_____
_____

DATE: _____

SEVERITY SCALE: 1 2 3 4 5 6 7 8 9 10

SYMPTOMS:
LIGHT SENSITIVITY: _   NAUSEA: _
SICKNESS: _   DIZZINESS: _
OTHER:_____

DURATION: _____

MEDICATION BEFORE MIGRAINE: _____
MEDICATION DURING MIGRAINE: _____
TREATMENT USED: _____
MOST EFFECTIVE TREATMENT: _____

TRIGGERS:
DIET 24 HOURS BEFORE MIGRAINE:
- FOOD: _____
- SNACKS: _____
- ALCOHOL: _____
- CAFFEINE: _____
- WATER: _____
- OTHER: _____

ODOURS: _____
STRESS: _____
CHANGES IN ROUTINE: _____
SLEEP PATTERN BEFORE MIGRAINE: _____
HORMONAL CHANGES (I.E. PERIOD): _____

POSSIBLE TRIGGERS FROM ABOVE INFORMATION: _____
NOTES: _____
_____
_____

DATE: _____

SEVERITY SCALE: 1 2 3 4 5 6 7 8 9 10

SYMPTOMS:
LIGHT SENSITIVITY: _   NAUSEA: _
SICKNESS: _   DIZZINESS: _
OTHER:_____

DURATION: _____

MEDICATION BEFORE MIGRAINE: _____
MEDICATION DURING MIGRAINE: _____
TREATMENT USED: _____
MOST EFFECTIVE TREATMENT: _____

TRIGGERS:
DIET 24 HOURS BEFORE MIGRAINE:
- FOOD: _____
- SNACKS: _____
- ALCOHOL: _____
- CAFFEINE: _____
- WATER: _____
- OTHER: _____

ODOURS: _____
STRESS: _____
CHANGES IN ROUTINE: _____
SLEEP PATTERN BEFORE MIGRAINE: _____
HORMONAL CHANGES (I.E. PERIOD): _____

POSSIBLE TRIGGERS FROM ABOVE INFORMATION: _____
NOTES: _____
_____
_____

DATE: _____

SEVERITY SCALE: 1 2 3 4 5 6 7 8 9 10

SYMPTOMS:
LIGHT SENSITIVITY: _   NAUSEA: _
SICKNESS: _   DIZZINESS: _
OTHER:_____

DURATION: _____

MEDICATION BEFORE MIGRAINE: _____
MEDICATION DURING MIGRAINE: _____
TREATMENT USED: _____
MOST EFFECTIVE TREATMENT: _____

TRIGGERS:
DIET 24 HOURS BEFORE MIGRAINE:
 - FOOD: _____
 - SNACKS: _____
 - ALCOHOL: _____
 - CAFFEINE: _____
 - WATER: _____
 - OTHER: _____

ODOURS: _____
STRESS: _____
CHANGES IN ROUTINE: _____
SLEEP PATTERN BEFORE MIGRAINE: _____
HORMONAL CHANGES (I.E. PERIOD): _____

POSSIBLE TRIGGERS FROM ABOVE INFORMATION: _____
NOTES: _____
_____
_____

DATE: _____

SEVERITY SCALE: 1 2 3 4 5 6 7 8 9 10

SYMPTOMS:
LIGHT SENSITIVITY: _   NAUSEA: _
SICKNESS: _   DIZZINESS: _
OTHER:_____

DURATION: _____

MEDICATION BEFORE MIGRAINE: _____
MEDICATION DURING MIGRAINE: _____
TREATMENT USED: _____
MOST EFFECTIVE TREATMENT: _____

TRIGGERS:
DIET 24 HOURS BEFORE MIGRAINE:
- FOOD: _____
- SNACKS: _____
- ALCOHOL: _____
- CAFFEINE: _____
- WATER: _____
- OTHER: _____

ODOURS: _____
STRESS: _____
CHANGES IN ROUTINE: _____
SLEEP PATTERN BEFORE MIGRAINE: _____
HORMONAL CHANGES (I.E. PERIOD): _____

POSSIBLE TRIGGERS FROM ABOVE INFORMATION: _____
NOTES: _____
_____
_____

DATE: _____

SEVERITY SCALE: 1 2 3 4 5 6 7 8 9 10

SYMPTOMS:
LIGHT SENSITIVITY: _   NAUSEA: _
SICKNESS: _   DIZZINESS: _
OTHER:_____

DURATION: _____

MEDICATION BEFORE MIGRAINE: _____
MEDICATION DURING MIGRAINE: _____
TREATMENT USED: _____
MOST EFFECTIVE TREATMENT: _____

TRIGGERS:
DIET 24 HOURS BEFORE MIGRAINE:
- FOOD: _____
- SNACKS: _____
- ALCOHOL: _____
- CAFFEINE: _____
- WATER: _____
- OTHER: _____

ODOURS: _____
STRESS: _____
CHANGES IN ROUTINE: _____
SLEEP PATTERN BEFORE MIGRAINE: _____
HORMONAL CHANGES (I.E. PERIOD): _____

POSSIBLE TRIGGERS FROM ABOVE INFORMATION: _____
NOTES: _____
_____
_____

DATE: _____

SEVERITY SCALE: 1 2 3 4 5 6 7 8 9 10

SYMPTOMS:
LIGHT SENSITIVITY: _   NAUSEA: _
SICKNESS: _   DIZZINESS: _
OTHER:_____

DURATION: _____

MEDICATION BEFORE MIGRAINE: _____
MEDICATION DURING MIGRAINE: _____
TREATMENT USED: _____
MOST EFFECTIVE TREATMENT: _____

TRIGGERS:
DIET 24 HOURS BEFORE MIGRAINE:
 - FOOD: _____
 - SNACKS: _____
 - ALCOHOL: _____
 - CAFFEINE: _____
 - WATER: _____
 - OTHER: _____

ODOURS: _____
STRESS: _____
CHANGES IN ROUTINE: _____
SLEEP PATTERN BEFORE MIGRAINE: _____
HORMONAL CHANGES (I.E. PERIOD): _____

POSSIBLE TRIGGERS FROM ABOVE INFORMATION: _____
NOTES: _____
_____
_____

DATE: _____

SEVERITY SCALE: 1 2 3 4 5 6 7 8 9 10

SYMPTOMS:
LIGHT SENSITIVITY: _   NAUSEA: _
SICKNESS: _   DIZZINESS: _
OTHER:_____

DURATION: _____

MEDICATION BEFORE MIGRAINE: _____
MEDICATION DURING MIGRAINE: _____
TREATMENT USED: _____
MOST EFFECTIVE TREATMENT: _____

TRIGGERS:
DIET 24 HOURS BEFORE MIGRAINE:
- FOOD: _____
- SNACKS: _____
- ALCOHOL: _____
- CAFFEINE: _____
- WATER: _____
- OTHER: _____

ODOURS: _____
STRESS: _____
CHANGES IN ROUTINE: _____
SLEEP PATTERN BEFORE MIGRAINE: _____
HORMONAL CHANGES (I.E. PERIOD): _____

POSSIBLE TRIGGERS FROM ABOVE INFORMATION: _____
NOTES: _____
_____
_____

DATE: _____

SEVERITY SCALE: 1 2 3 4 5 6 7 8 9 10

SYMPTOMS:
LIGHT SENSITIVITY: _   NAUSEA: _
SICKNESS: _   DIZZINESS: _
OTHER:_____

DURATION: _____

MEDICATION BEFORE MIGRAINE: _____
MEDICATION DURING MIGRAINE: _____
TREATMENT USED: _____
MOST EFFECTIVE TREATMENT: _____

TRIGGERS:
DIET 24 HOURS BEFORE MIGRAINE:
- FOOD: _____
- SNACKS: _____
- ALCOHOL: _____
- CAFFEINE: _____
- WATER: _____
- OTHER: _____

ODOURS: _____
STRESS: _____
CHANGES IN ROUTINE: _____
SLEEP PATTERN BEFORE MIGRAINE: _____
HORMONAL CHANGES (I.E. PERIOD): _____

POSSIBLE TRIGGERS FROM ABOVE INFORMATION: _____
NOTES: _____
_____
_____

DATE: _____

SEVERITY SCALE: 1 2 3 4 5 6 7 8 9 10

SYMPTOMS:
LIGHT SENSITIVITY: _   NAUSEA: _
SICKNESS: _   DIZZINESS: _
OTHER:_____

DURATION: _____

MEDICATION BEFORE MIGRAINE: _____
MEDICATION DURING MIGRAINE: _____
TREATMENT USED: _____
MOST EFFECTIVE TREATMENT: _____

TRIGGERS:
DIET 24 HOURS BEFORE MIGRAINE:
- FOOD: _____
- SNACKS: _____
- ALCOHOL: _____
- CAFFEINE: _____
- WATER: _____
- OTHER: _____

ODOURS: _____
STRESS: _____
CHANGES IN ROUTINE: _____
SLEEP PATTERN BEFORE MIGRAINE: _____
HORMONAL CHANGES (I.E. PERIOD): _____

POSSIBLE TRIGGERS FROM ABOVE INFORMATION: _____
NOTES: _____
_____
_____

DATE: _____

SEVERITY SCALE: 1 2 3 4 5 6 7 8 9 10

SYMPTOMS:
LIGHT SENSITIVITY: _   NAUSEA: _
SICKNESS: _   DIZZINESS: _
OTHER:_____

DURATION: _____

MEDICATION BEFORE MIGRAINE: _____
MEDICATION DURING MIGRAINE: _____
TREATMENT USED: _____
MOST EFFECTIVE TREATMENT: _____

TRIGGERS:
DIET 24 HOURS BEFORE MIGRAINE:
- FOOD: _____
- SNACKS: _____
- ALCOHOL: _____
- CAFFEINE: _____
- WATER: _____
- OTHER: _____

ODOURS: _____
STRESS: _____
CHANGES IN ROUTINE: _____
SLEEP PATTERN BEFORE MIGRAINE: _____
HORMONAL CHANGES (I.E. PERIOD): _____

POSSIBLE TRIGGERS FROM ABOVE INFORMATION: _____
NOTES: _____
_____
_____

DATE: _____

SEVERITY SCALE: 1 2 3 4 5 6 7 8 9 10

SYMPTOMS:
LIGHT SENSITIVITY: _   NAUSEA: _
SICKNESS: _   DIZZINESS: _
OTHER:_____

DURATION: _____

MEDICATION BEFORE MIGRAINE: _____
MEDICATION DURING MIGRAINE: _____
TREATMENT USED: _____
MOST EFFECTIVE TREATMENT: _____

TRIGGERS:
DIET 24 HOURS BEFORE MIGRAINE:
- FOOD: _____
- SNACKS: _____
- ALCOHOL: _____
- CAFFEINE: _____
- WATER: _____
- OTHER: _____

ODOURS: _____
STRESS: _____
CHANGES IN ROUTINE: _____
SLEEP PATTERN BEFORE MIGRAINE: _____
HORMONAL CHANGES (I.E. PERIOD): _____

POSSIBLE TRIGGERS FROM ABOVE INFORMATION: _____
NOTES: _____
_____
_____

DATE: _____

SEVERITY SCALE: 1 2 3 4 5 6 7 8 9 10

SYMPTOMS:
LIGHT SENSITIVITY: _   NAUSEA: _
SICKNESS: _   DIZZINESS: _
OTHER:_____

DURATION: _____

MEDICATION BEFORE MIGRAINE: _____
MEDICATION DURING MIGRAINE: _____
TREATMENT USED: _____
MOST EFFECTIVE TREATMENT: _____

TRIGGERS:
DIET 24 HOURS BEFORE MIGRAINE:
- FOOD: _____
- SNACKS: _____
- ALCOHOL: _____
- CAFFEINE: _____
- WATER: _____
- OTHER: _____

ODOURS: _____
STRESS: _____
CHANGES IN ROUTINE: _____
SLEEP PATTERN BEFORE MIGRAINE: _____
HORMONAL CHANGES (I.E. PERIOD): _____

POSSIBLE TRIGGERS FROM ABOVE INFORMATION: _____
NOTES: _____
_____
_____

DATE: _____

SEVERITY SCALE: 1 2 3 4 5 6 7 8 9 10

SYMPTOMS:
LIGHT SENSITIVITY: _   NAUSEA: _
SICKNESS: _   DIZZINESS: _
OTHER:_____

DURATION: _____

MEDICATION BEFORE MIGRAINE: _____
MEDICATION DURING MIGRAINE: _____
TREATMENT USED: _____
MOST EFFECTIVE TREATMENT: _____

TRIGGERS:
DIET 24 HOURS BEFORE MIGRAINE:
- FOOD: _____
- SNACKS: _____
- ALCOHOL: _____
- CAFFEINE: _____
- WATER: _____
- OTHER: _____

ODOURS: _____
STRESS: _____
CHANGES IN ROUTINE: _____
SLEEP PATTERN BEFORE MIGRAINE: _____
HORMONAL CHANGES (I.E. PERIOD): _____

POSSIBLE TRIGGERS FROM ABOVE INFORMATION: _____
NOTES: _____
_____
_____

DATE: _____

SEVERITY SCALE: 1 2 3 4 5 6 7 8 9 10

SYMPTOMS:
LIGHT SENSITIVITY: _   NAUSEA: _
SICKNESS: _   DIZZINESS: _
OTHER:_____

DURATION: _____

MEDICATION BEFORE MIGRAINE: _____
MEDICATION DURING MIGRAINE: _____
TREATMENT USED: _____
MOST EFFECTIVE TREATMENT: _____

TRIGGERS:
DIET 24 HOURS BEFORE MIGRAINE:
- FOOD: _____
- SNACKS: _____
- ALCOHOL: _____
- CAFFEINE: _____
- WATER: _____
- OTHER: _____

ODOURS: _____
STRESS: _____
CHANGES IN ROUTINE: _____
SLEEP PATTERN BEFORE MIGRAINE: _____
HORMONAL CHANGES (I.E. PERIOD): _____

POSSIBLE TRIGGERS FROM ABOVE INFORMATION: _____
NOTES: _____
_____
_____

DATE: _____

SEVERITY SCALE: 1 2 3 4 5 6 7 8 9 10

SYMPTOMS:
LIGHT SENSITIVITY: _   NAUSEA: _
SICKNESS: _   DIZZINESS: _
OTHER:_____

DURATION: _____

MEDICATION BEFORE MIGRAINE: _____
MEDICATION DURING MIGRAINE: _____
TREATMENT USED: _____
MOST EFFECTIVE TREATMENT: _____

TRIGGERS:
DIET 24 HOURS BEFORE MIGRAINE:
- FOOD: _____
- SNACKS: _____
- ALCOHOL: _____
- CAFFEINE: _____
- WATER: _____
- OTHER: _____

ODOURS: _____
STRESS: _____
CHANGES IN ROUTINE: _____
SLEEP PATTERN BEFORE MIGRAINE: _____
HORMONAL CHANGES (I.E. PERIOD): _____

POSSIBLE TRIGGERS FROM ABOVE INFORMATION: _____
NOTES: _____
_____
_____

DATE: _____

SEVERITY SCALE: 1 2 3 4 5 6 7 8 9 10

SYMPTOMS:
LIGHT SENSITIVITY: _   NAUSEA: _
SICKNESS: _   DIZZINESS: _
OTHER:_____

DURATION: _____

MEDICATION BEFORE MIGRAINE: _____
MEDICATION DURING MIGRAINE: _____
TREATMENT USED: _____
MOST EFFECTIVE TREATMENT: _____

TRIGGERS:
DIET 24 HOURS BEFORE MIGRAINE:
- FOOD: _____
- SNACKS: _____
- ALCOHOL: _____
- CAFFEINE: _____
- WATER: _____
- OTHER: _____

ODOURS: _____
STRESS: _____
CHANGES IN ROUTINE: _____
SLEEP PATTERN BEFORE MIGRAINE: _____
HORMONAL CHANGES (I.E. PERIOD): _____

POSSIBLE TRIGGERS FROM ABOVE INFORMATION: _____
NOTES: _____
_____
_____

DATE: _____

SEVERITY SCALE: 1 2 3 4 5 6 7 8 9 10

SYMPTOMS:
LIGHT SENSITIVITY: _   NAUSEA: _
SICKNESS: _   DIZZINESS: _
OTHER:_____

DURATION: _____

MEDICATION BEFORE MIGRAINE: _____
MEDICATION DURING MIGRAINE: _____
TREATMENT USED: _____
MOST EFFECTIVE TREATMENT: _____

TRIGGERS:
DIET 24 HOURS BEFORE MIGRAINE:
- FOOD: _____
- SNACKS: _____
- ALCOHOL: _____
- CAFFEINE: _____
- WATER: _____
- OTHER: _____

ODOURS: _____
STRESS: _____
CHANGES IN ROUTINE: _____
SLEEP PATTERN BEFORE MIGRAINE: _____
HORMONAL CHANGES (I.E. PERIOD): _____

POSSIBLE TRIGGERS FROM ABOVE INFORMATION: _____
NOTES: _____
_____
_____

DATE: _____

SEVERITY SCALE: 1 2 3 4 5 6 7 8 9 10

SYMPTOMS:
LIGHT SENSITIVITY: _   NAUSEA: _
SICKNESS: _   DIZZINESS: _
OTHER:_____

DURATION: _____

MEDICATION BEFORE MIGRAINE: _____
MEDICATION DURING MIGRAINE: _____
TREATMENT USED: _____
MOST EFFECTIVE TREATMENT: _____

TRIGGERS:
DIET 24 HOURS BEFORE MIGRAINE:
- FOOD: _____
- SNACKS: _____
- ALCOHOL: _____
- CAFFEINE: _____
- WATER: _____
- OTHER: _____

ODOURS: _____
STRESS: _____
CHANGES IN ROUTINE: _____
SLEEP PATTERN BEFORE MIGRAINE: _____
HORMONAL CHANGES (I.E. PERIOD): _____

POSSIBLE TRIGGERS FROM ABOVE INFORMATION: _____
NOTES: _____
_____
_____

DATE: _____

SEVERITY SCALE: 1 2 3 4 5 6 7 8 9 10

SYMPTOMS:
LIGHT SENSITIVITY: _   NAUSEA: _
SICKNESS: _   DIZZINESS: _
OTHER:_____

DURATION: _____

MEDICATION BEFORE MIGRAINE: _____
MEDICATION DURING MIGRAINE: _____
TREATMENT USED: _____
MOST EFFECTIVE TREATMENT: _____

TRIGGERS:
DIET 24 HOURS BEFORE MIGRAINE:
- FOOD: _____
- SNACKS: _____
- ALCOHOL: _____
- CAFFEINE: _____
- WATER: _____
- OTHER: _____

ODOURS: _____
STRESS: _____
CHANGES IN ROUTINE: _____
SLEEP PATTERN BEFORE MIGRAINE: _____
HORMONAL CHANGES (I.E. PERIOD): _____

POSSIBLE TRIGGERS FROM ABOVE INFORMATION: _____
NOTES: _____
_____
_____

DATE: _____

SEVERITY SCALE: 1 2 3 4 5 6 7 8 9 10

SYMPTOMS:
LIGHT SENSITIVITY: _   NAUSEA: _
SICKNESS: _   DIZZINESS: _
OTHER:_____

DURATION: _____

MEDICATION BEFORE MIGRAINE: _____
MEDICATION DURING MIGRAINE: _____
TREATMENT USED: _____
MOST EFFECTIVE TREATMENT: _____

TRIGGERS:
DIET 24 HOURS BEFORE MIGRAINE:
 - FOOD: _____
 - SNACKS: _____
 - ALCOHOL: _____
 - CAFFEINE: _____
 - WATER: _____
 - OTHER: _____

ODOURS: _____
STRESS: _____
CHANGES IN ROUTINE: _____
SLEEP PATTERN BEFORE MIGRAINE: _____
HORMONAL CHANGES (I.E. PERIOD): _____

POSSIBLE TRIGGERS FROM ABOVE INFORMATION: _____
NOTES: _____
_____
_____

MONTHLY REVIEW:

MONTH: _____

NUMBER OF MIGRAINES: _____

NUMBER OF MOST SEVERE MIGRAINES: _____

NUMBER OF DAYS I HAD A MIGRAINE: _____

REPEATING TRIGGERS: _____

IS THERE A PATTERN/CYCLE WHEN MIGRAINE IS MOST LIKELY TO OCCUR?

_____

_____

MOST EFFECTIVE TREATMENT? _____

CHANGES TO IMPLEMENT, BASED ON THE ABOVE? _____

_____

NOTES/OBSERVATIONS: _____

_____

_____

_____

_____

MONTHLY REVIEW:

MONTH: _____

NUMBER OF MIGRAINES: _____

NUMBER OF MOST SEVERE MIGRAINES: _____

NUMBER OF DAYS I HAD A MIGRAINE: _____

REPEATING TRIGGERS: _____

IS THERE A PATTERN/CYCLE WHEN MIGRAINE IS MOST LIKELY TO OCCUR?

_____

_____

MOST EFFECTIVE TREATMENT? _____

CHANGES TO IMPLEMENT, BASED ON THE ABOVE? _____

_____

NOTES/OBSERVATIONS: _____

_____

_____

_____

_____

MONTHLY REVIEW:

MONTH: _____

NUMBER OF MIGRAINES: _____

NUMBER OF MOST SEVERE MIGRAINES: _____

NUMBER OF DAYS I HAD A MIGRAINE: _____

REPEATING TRIGGERS: _____

IS THERE A PATTERN/CYCLE WHEN MIGRAINE IS MOST LIKELY TO OCCUR?

_____

_____

MOST EFFECTIVE TREATMENT? _____

CHANGES TO IMPLEMENT, BASED ON THE ABOVE? _____

_____

NOTES/OBSERVATIONS: _____

_____

_____

_____

MONTHLY REVIEW:

MONTH: _____

NUMBER OF MIGRAINES: _____

NUMBER OF MOST SEVERE MIGRAINES: _____

NUMBER OF DAYS I HAD A MIGRAINE: _____

REPEATING TRIGGERS: _____

IS THERE A PATTERN/CYCLE WHEN MIGRAINE IS MOST LIKELY TO OCCUR?

_____

_____

MOST EFFECTIVE TREATMENT? _____

CHANGES TO IMPLEMENT, BASED ON THE ABOVE? _____

_____

NOTES/OBSERVATIONS: _____

_____

_____

_____

_____

MONTHLY REVIEW:

MONTH: _____

NUMBER OF MIGRAINES: _____

NUMBER OF MOST SEVERE MIGRAINES: _____

NUMBER OF DAYS I HAD A MIGRAINE: _____

REPEATING TRIGGERS: _____

IS THERE A PATTERN/CYCLE WHEN MIGRAINE IS MOST LIKELY TO OCCUR?

_____

_____

MOST EFFECTIVE TREATMENT? _____

CHANGES TO IMPLEMENT, BASED ON THE ABOVE? _____

_____

NOTES/OBSERVATIONS: _____

_____

_____

_____

_____

MONTHLY REVIEW:

MONTH: _____

NUMBER OF MIGRAINES: _____

NUMBER OF MOST SEVERE MIGRAINES: _____

NUMBER OF DAYS I HAD A MIGRAINE: _____

REPEATING TRIGGERS: _____

IS THERE A PATTERN/CYCLE WHEN MIGRAINE IS MOST LIKELY TO OCCUR?

_____

_____

MOST EFFECTIVE TREATMENT? _____

CHANGES TO IMPLEMENT, BASED ON THE ABOVE? _____

_____

NOTES/OBSERVATIONS: _____

_____

_____

_____

_____

MONTHLY REVIEW:

MONTH: _____

NUMBER OF MIGRAINES: _____

NUMBER OF MOST SEVERE MIGRAINES: _____

NUMBER OF DAYS I HAD A MIGRAINE: _____

REPEATING TRIGGERS: _____

IS THERE A PATTERN/CYCLE WHEN MIGRAINE IS MOST LIKELY TO OCCUR?

_____

_____

MOST EFFECTIVE TREATMENT? _____

CHANGES TO IMPLEMENT, BASED ON THE ABOVE? _____

_____

NOTES/OBSERVATIONS: _____

_____

_____

_____

_____

MONTHLY REVIEW:

MONTH: _____

NUMBER OF MIGRAINES: _____

NUMBER OF MOST SEVERE MIGRAINES: _____

NUMBER OF DAYS I HAD A MIGRAINE: _____

REPEATING TRIGGERS: _____

IS THERE A PATTERN/CYCLE WHEN MIGRAINE IS MOST LIKELY TO OCCUR?

_____

_____

MOST EFFECTIVE TREATMENT? _____

CHANGES TO IMPLEMENT, BASED ON THE ABOVE? _____

_____

NOTES/OBSERVATIONS: _____

_____

_____

_____

_____

NOTES: